What others are saying

"Play bald! Dave Beswick proves that a positive attitude and a sense of humor more than equal the most elegantly coifed head."
— Pete Van Wieren, Atlanta Braves Broadcaster

"Dave Beswick's research and data are very evident in his new winner about the bald dome."
— Dick Vitale, ESPN Sports

"Dave Beswick is a true brother of the bald. We are proud to be on the same team with him in promoting a positive image and the acceptance of baldness. If you are using more draino than shampoo and want to make real headway, read this inspiring and humorful book."
— John T. Capps III, Founder of the Bald-Headed Men of America

"Dave Beswick scratched his head again and came up with another fun book of humorous short stories, jokes, cartoons, historical notes, and a few serious comments about the millions of men and women blessed with an abundance of barren real estate between their ears."
— Sam Venable, Knoxville News-Sentinel

"This humorous and insightful book will help anyone more fully understand and appreciate bald men everywhere."
— Ty Koontz, author of *Underwater Sunlight*

"So what'll it be, locks or a bagel? After reading this book I've decided to leave my pate in place."
— Pat Thompson, probation officer, counselor

What others are saying about this book:

"As an investment counselor I'm always encouraging people to pay off their debts and save money. After reading this book I now see how bald men can save money by not spending it on haircuts and hair care products. Saving around $327.00 a year is a good head start."
— Rosemary Gilliam, Merrill Lynch Assistant
Vice-President and Senior Financial Consultant

"The new bald vocabulary is a definite dome improvement raising cranial nudity to new levels of respectability. 'Cue ball' and 'follicly challenged' are now 'sculptured speed bump' and 'follicly natural.' The hair-free Daniel Webster would be proud!"
— Jerry Seitz, Academic Dean of Kennedy
High School in Seattle, WA

"Once you start a second face, this book can lead you to hair peace on the other side of hair."
— Bob Tallon, co-author of
The Enneagram at Work

Bald Men Never Have a Bad Hair Day

Wit and Wisdom
for Men on the Bald Path

Dave Beswick

Ama Publishing

St. Augustine, Florida

Bald Men Never Have a Bad Hair Day

Wit and Wisdom
for Men on the Bald Path

by Dave Beswick

Published by: **Ama Publishing**
Post Office Box 840117
St. Augustine Beach, FL. 32084-0117 U.S.A.

Printed in the United States of America

Illustrations by Kurt Snibbe

ISBN 0-9613176-2-0

LCCN 97-94685

Acknowledgments

Imagine having your best friend, wife, proofreader, and intuitive critic at your beck and call. Janie is all of these talents rolled into one spiced with spontaneous humor, love, and a bucketful of back rubs. After Janie reviewed the material, her words, "I like it," "take it out," "sleep on it," or "go for a swim and something will come," kept the book and me moving forward in a positive way. If I am the Captain of Chrome, then she is the best first mate anyone could have.

Thank you, John T. Capps, for your friendship, bald resources, and wonderful sense of humor. And to you, Jane Capps; your friendship and hospitality warm our hearts.

Thanks, Kurt Snibbe, for making the book come alive with your original, witty, and uplifting illustrations.

Our friends keep the ship afloat during times of navigating to and fro. Many thanks to the Harraka family for opening their home to us in New Jersey. And for allowing us to relax and work out in Knoxville, Tennessee, thank you Carolyn Gentry. And a special "Helloooo Janet!" to Janet Lydecker whose constant support gives wind to our sails.

Cover layout and design by Regine De Toledo of Graphics Ink. Book design and typography by Chris Nolt of Cirrus Design. Editing by Stacey Lynn. Book printed by Patterson Printing.

Guys with hair are overdressed.
— *Carl Reiner*

Contents

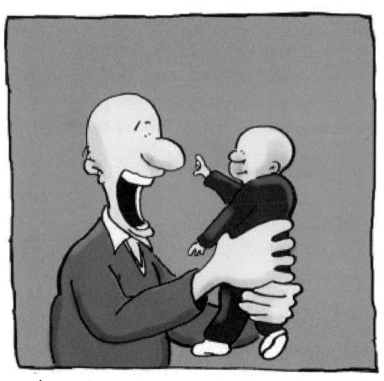

YEAH, WE HAVE THE SAME HAIRCUT!

Introduction

Bald Men Never Have a Bad Hair Day is the second book in the "Bald Men" series. Taking up where Bald Men Always Come Out on Top left off, it carries on the proud salute to the 40 million bald men in the United States and some 432 million more worldwide.

You will benefit from this book if:

- You are looking into the various options to hair loss and want to consider the advantages of learning to accept what you have and make the most of it.

- You are happily hairless and want to learn more creative things you can say and do relative to your head to spread joy and laughter wherever you go.

- You know or love a baldheaded man and want to give him a book that says, "You're the best!"

In the first chapter, "It's in the Genes Baby!" you will learn about the discovery of the first human gene associated with hair loss, what the prospects are for future hair-raising developments, and important questions to consider before investing in rugs, plugs, drugs, or future bald gene treatments. You will also learn why millions of men enjoy their pearly pates and wouldn't think of covering up, even if the bald gene could be altered to grow hair.

How do you know when you're going bald?

Chapter 2 gives you all the clues. For example, you know you're going bald when it takes longer to wash your face and your dandruff has completely disappeared. Use any of these 30 responses whenever you are asked the question, "When did you first start losing your hair?" and you will bring humor to bare in any situation.

Millions of wonderful bald men have gone before us and left a legacy more rich and valuable than hair will ever be. By honoring and appreciating what these men have given to our world, we say "yes" to ourselves and the unique gifts that we have to contribute. Chapter 3 presents 108 follicly natural artists, writers, leaders, entertainers, musicians, politicians, social activists, and sports figures who have paved the way smooth for the rest of us. Now, it is our turn to gain strength from these men whose lives inspire us to follow our hearts and dreams. You will also learn about the Bald-Headed Men of America, a benevolent organization that honors these bald men and promotes acceptance and making the most of what you have.

An important ingredient in coming to accept and appreciate our bald heads is to recognize the many advantages that a topless testosterone top has to offer. "Baldness Increases Your Face Value: The Advantages of Being Bald" offers 39 perks of being bald and clearly conveys the message that being hair-free is a wonderful and even preferable way to be.

Why did God allow men to go bald in the first place? Why wasn't everyone allowed to have hair for a lifetime? Are there barbershops in heaven? In chapter 5,

God answers these and other key questions about baldness from a celestine perspective.

Chapter 6 tells you 48 things that bald golfers know so that you can have a bagful of witty things to say when you hit the links with your friends. For example, bald golfers know that bald heads are "Taylor made" by God and that for discerning women, a man's bald head is a fairway to heaven.

Chapter 7, "Hair Ye, Hair Ye, What Is Thy Purpose?" presents a hair analysis of how the purpose of hair has changed from caveman days to the present.

When having guests over it's fun to play trivia games. With "Bald Trivia II" you have 55 questions that are guaranteed to elicit laughter as well as inform your guests of some of the great bald men and the contributions they have made to the world. It's another great way to use your head to bring good cheer and a positive bald experience to any gathering. By keeping score and offering prizes for the winners, you create a lightly competitive atmosphere that adds to the fun.

Chapter 9, "The Eagle Has Landed: Societal Acceptance of Baldness Close at Hand," provides us with a history of the most influential barren beacons from 1950 to the present. All of these eagle scouts have paved the way for the Eagle who was to come. The great bird of flight has finally landed and changed the face of thousands of heads around the world. With a train of esteemed bald men leading to the Head Engine, this man has made baldness a headstyle that shows no signs of receding.

As millions of men are proudly and voluntarily

donning the dynamic dome, the time is ripe to change the way we think and speak about the sacred space known as our head. "Dome Improvement: A New Vocabulary for the Emerging Bald Paradigm" teaches bald men and those who love them a new vocabulary aimed at replacing all derogatory words formerly used to describe baldheaded men. For example, if someone calls us "cue ball" or "bowling ball" we need to inform them that these words have been replaced with "sculptured speed bump" and "rolling stone."

In Chapter 11, "The Bald Path: A Smooth Road in a Rocky World," we learn what the Bald Path is and the values of Bald Pathers who choose to walk in harmony with bald men, women, and children everywhere.

We hope you enjoy this book and that it will inspire you to take plenty of time to appreciate and enjoy your beautiful bald head. May it be a source of joy for you and those you meet along the way.

It's in the Genes Baby!

Scientists have been claiming for years that the cause and "cure" for hair loss is in the genes. In response, balding comedian George Carlin said, "I don't know what the big fuss is all about. I've looked in my jeans plenty of times and found no hair loss whatsoever!"

For decades scientists have been looking for the illusive bald gene, that when set loose, could turn on the switch for growing hair. Then, in their January, 1998 press release, researchers at Columbia University College of Physicians and Surgeons announced that they literally flipped their wigs when they saw the first human gene associated with hair loss glaring at them right in the face. Like excited parents having given birth to their first child, they couldn't help but name their newborn. "Hairless" was the appellation they chose. Perhaps "Seymore Hair" would've been more appropriate, but it's not worth splitting hairs over.

It used to be that if you had the bald gene, then what you had was a permanent wave good-bye. Like the leopard that could not change its spots, if you had the bald gene no amount of massaging, praying, taking vitamins, or using scalp lotions or medications could restore the fuzz that was. But now, the bald truth about the bald gene *may* be changing.

This bald gene discovery *may* be the scientific breakthrough that leads to hair-raising developments. On the other end, it may not cause anybody's hair to stand on end or even lay flat. In the meantime we encourage every bald(ing) man to consider this maxim: *Peace of mind is the ability to accept what is and make the most of it.* Also, we invite him to examine these core questions before deciding which alternative to hair loss is right for him: Is having hair on my head essential to living a happy, love-filled, and successful life? What are my options (i.e., a combover, toupee, hair weave, hair growth medication, scalp reduction, hair lift, micro-graftings, the future bald gene treatment) and why am I *really* considering getting a hair addition? (Note: if you're doing it to get loved or to avoid rejection, the new addition will not do it for you.) We encourage you to not only consider the standard alternatives to hair loss, but also to ponder the benefits of accepting and making the most of what you have as a viable option.

What are some of the benefits of saying "yes" to our barren beacons? For starters, the fact is that right now millions of discriminating women are baldhead-over-heels in love with maneless men.

They simply like the way the bald head looks, the way it feels, and appreciate having more open space to kiss and caress. Being topless saves an average of three days a year normally spent combing, washing, blow drying and getting the hairs just right, and over $300 a year on haircuts, shampoo, brushes and the like. Hair-free men never have to worry what others are thinking about their combover or new hair addition, or which way they're facing in the wind. They stay looking the same age for a long period of time, are always neat and wrinkle-free, and never have a bad hair day. And perhaps best of all, when company comes over all they have to do is straighten their shirt.

These men know that good comedians get a lot of laughs whenever they joke about a particular part of their anatomy. Thus, they choose to use their heads as an asset to bring joy and laughter to others. As an added benefit, every time they flaunt their threadbare epidermis for the sake of others' enjoyment, they feel even better about themselves and their solar powered peaks.

How exactly do these topless men use their heads? For instance, when asked, "How are you?" they can reply, "Great! I was just elected the head of the Skin Club for Men." They can also ask people bald trivia questions like: Bald monks are aerodynamically designed to go straight to heaven. True or false? Answer: True. And, by asking for an estimate at a barber shop and explaining to people that their hair didn't really fall out, it just went underground and came out their nose and ears, they will appreciate the smiles and laughter they receive in return.

Through our books and the Bald-Headed Men of America, we promote the least expensive, least worrisome, and least painful option to hair loss there is—namely, acceptance and making the most of what you have with a healthy dose of humor thrown in. We strive to help people realize that baldness is not a disease, that needs to be cured. Rather, it is a choice, a positive headstyle that provides individuals with a unique and distinctive alternative.

At this moment in time, thousands of men on mother earth have voluntarily shaved their heads. Why? Following the lead of professional athletes, actors, musicians, and world and spiritual leaders, it offers a way for individuals to be different and to get a headstart on the wave of the future. Also, the naked noggin is smooth and sexy and requires very low maintenance. It is a no-stress hairstyle since you don't need mirrors and don't have to be constantly checking your hair to make sure it looks good or is in place. It gives you a certain look of authority in the workplace and reflects clean living and no faking. And finally, when you lean over to make that all-important putt in golf, hair will never fall into your eyes.

You Know You Are Going
Bald When . . .

One of the most frequently asked questions of those of us with clean slates is, "When did you first start losing your hair?" Rather than respond in the usual manner by giving a particular age or time period in our life, we now have 30 witty things we can say to add humor to any situation. For instance, we can answer: "I knew that I was going bald when flies started using my head as a landing strip. And it really hit home when I was voted most likely to recede at my high school graduation."

You know you are going bald when . . .

- It takes longer to wash your face.
- You're the first one to hear snowflakes.
- You only press the cool button when using the hair dryer.
- Your comb is hairier than your head.

You know you're going bald when. . .

- Your barber talks more than he cuts.
- You receive an invitation to attend the annual *Bald-Headed Men of America Convention*.
- Flies start using your head as a landing strip.
- You watch a late-night hair replacement ad from start to finish.
- You overhear your small son tell the barber: "I want a haircut like my daddy's—with a hole on top."
- You start growing facial hair or a ponytail.
- You have a parting of the waves.
- You go from being vain to seeing vein.
- You wonder why your parents didn't name you Seymore Head.
- Someone tells you that you have a very nicely shaped head.
- You are down to the bare essentials.
- You notice that a hair on your head is worth two in the brush.
- Your friends tell you that you were easy to spot in the dark theater.
- You make a truck flap arrangement out of your side hairs and flip them over the open space.

You know you're going bald when. . .

- Your baseball hat becomes part of your daily wardrobe.
- You carry fewer bottles with you into the shower.
- You style your hair by pushing it rather than brushing it.
- You are voted most likely to recede at your high school graduation.
- You ask for an estimate before choosing your barber.
- You wipe 'n go after eating spicy foods.
- You stand on your toes or get elevator shoes so that people will look you straight in the eye rather than focus on your hairline.
- You receive a soft cotton nightcap to keep your head warm as a gift from a loved one.
- A "friend" asks you, "Who parted your hair, Moses?"
- The hairballs in your bathroom get smaller and smaller.
- Women stare at you because they've heard that bald men don't use their hormones for growing hair.
- Your dandruff disappears completely.

Ours is the only organization that grows
because of lack of growth. We believe that
skin is in and if you don't have it, flaunt it.
— *John T. Capps III, founder*
of the Bald-Headed Men
of America

Famous Bald Men:
Shining Stars Past and Present

Millions of wonderful bald men have gone before us and left a legacy more rich and valuable than hair will ever be. By honoring and appreciating what these men have given to our world, we affirm ourselves and the unique gifts we have to contribute. The following is a list of 108 follicly natural artists, writers, leaders, entertainers, musicians, politicians, social activists, and sports figures who have paved the way smooth for the rest of us. Now it is our turn to gain strength from these men who have shown clearly that hair is not necessary to make a positive and lasting contribution to the world.

For the shining stars in the movies and world of sports, who give us needed escape from our daily rounds of obligations, we are grateful. For the Brylcreemless comedians who provide us much to laugh about, we smile in appreciation. For our lustrous political and spiritual leaders who have chosen not to cover up but to be beacons of light for the sake of the greater good, we give our regard. To the waveless writers and teachers on the cutting edge of new ideas, we say "thank you" for calling us to open our minds and to think in new, loving, and inclusive ways. And to the smooth musicians and artists: our souls have been massaged by your touch of graceful creativity.

Actors, Entertainers, Producers

Robert Duvall	*Actor*
Mickey Rooney	*Actor*
Bruce Willis	*Actor*
Harpo Marx	*Comedian*
Don Rickles	*Comedian, actor*
Zero Mostel	*Comedian, actor*
Dom DeLuise	*Comedian, actor*
W. C. Fields	*Comedian, actor*
Walter Brennan	*TV actor on "The Real McCoys"*
Richard Moll	*TV actor, shaved bailiff on "Night Court"*
Art Carney	*TV actor, sidekick on "Jackie Gleason Show"*
William Frawley	*TV actor, neighbor in "I Love Lucy"*
Allen Funt	*TV host of "Candid Camera"*
Charles Kuralt	*TV journalist*

Burl Ives	*Singer, actor*
P. T. Barnum	*American showman*
Alfred Hitchcock	*British-American film director*
Otto Preminger	*Film director*
Norman Lear	*TV producer*

World Leaders

Chiang Kai-shek	*Chinese political leader*
Helmut Kohl	*German chancellor*
David Ben-Gurion	*Israeli prime minister*
Demetrios Maximos	*Minister of Greece*
Benito Mussolini	*Italian dictator*
Ho Chi Minh	*Vietnamese leader, revolutionary*
Giuseppi Garibaldi	*Italian military leader*
Otto Von Bismarck	*Prussian statesman*
Zenko Suziki	*Japanese prime minister*
Georges Clemenceu	*French premier*

Writers, Artists, Musicians

Bernie Siegel	*Author of* Love, Medicine, and Miracles
Ken Wilber	*Author,* New Age philosopher

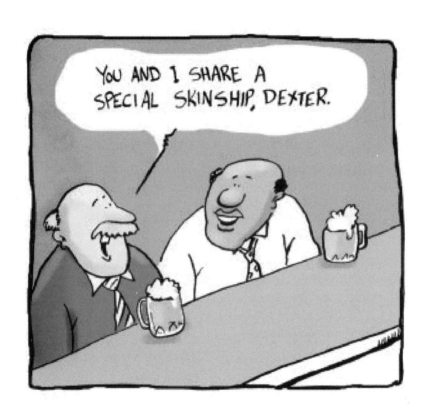

Hans Christian Anderson	*Danish writer*
Art Buchwald	*Columnist*
Thomas Hardy	*British novelist, poet, architect*
Alfred, Lord Tennyson	*English poet*
Truman Capote	*Novelist*
Socrates	*Greek philosopher*
Voltaire	*Poet, dramatist*
Leo Tolstoy	*Novelist and philosopher*
Henry Mancini	*Oscar-winning composer, musician, songwriter*
Arthur Toscanini	*Conductor*
Peter Ilich Tchaikovsky	*Composer*
James Taylor	*Singer and songwriter*
Peter Yarrow	*Folksinger*
Paul Stookey	*Folksinger*
Frank Lloyd Wright	*Architect*
Ravi Shankar	*Indian sitarist*
Count Basie	*Pianist*
Art Garfunkel	*Singer*
Arthur Murray	*Dance instructor*

Social/Political Figures

Ed Koch	*Mayor of New York*
Ben Franklin	*Inventor*
Douglas MacArthur	*U.S. military leader*
Alexander Haig Jr.	*U.S. Secretary of State*
Jacob Javits	*U.S. senator*
Alan Cranston	*U.S. senator*
Andrew Carnegie	*Industrialist and philanthropist*
Suleyman Demirel	*Turkish political leader*
Melvin Laird	*U.S. representative*
Jacques Piccard	*Ocean explorer*
Moshe Dayan	*Israeli statesman*
Sam Walton	*Wal-Mart founder*
Keith Robert Murdock	*Businessman, publisher*
Chuck Yeager	*Test pilot*
Alan Bean	*Astronaut*
Charles Lindberg	*Aviator*

Spiritual Figures

Ram Das	*Spiritual leader, author*
Cardinal Spellman	*Wrote* The Road to Victory
Reinhold Niebuhr	*Protestant theologian*
Dalai Lama	*Buddhist leader, Nobel Peace Prize winner*

Sports Figures

Evander Holyfield	*Boxer*
Mark Messier	*Hockey player, a quintessential gladiator*
Dennis Hull	*Hockey wing*
Scotty Bowman	*Hockey coach, won 3 Stanley Cups*
Ivan Johnson	*Hockey defenseman*
Jim Brown	*Football running back*
Paul Hornung	*Football player*
John Riggins	*Football running back*
Garo Yepremian	*Football kicker*
Max McGee	*Football receiver*
Fred Biletnifoff	*Football receiver*
Ray Nitschke	*Football linebacker (number 66)*
Otis Sistrunk	*Football lineman*
Mel Renfro	*Football defensive back*
Herb Adderly	*Football defensive back*
George Halas	*Football head coach*
Harmon Killebrew	*Baseball player in the Hall of Fame*
Vic Power	*Baseball player*
Matt Williams	*Baseball player*
Enos Slaughter	*Baseball player*

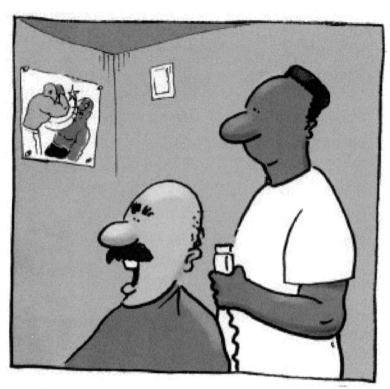

GIVE ME THE HOLYFIELD HAIRCUT, BUT WATCH THE EARS.

Gaylord Perry	*Baseball pitcher, winner of the Cy Young award*
Warren Spahn	*Baseball pitcher in the Hall of Fame*
Cy Young	*Baseball pitcher*
Eddie Matthews	*Baseball player, hit over 500 home runs*
Leo Durocher	*Baseball player, manager, Hall of Famer*
Walter Alston	*Baseball manager*
Sean McDonough	*Baseball/college football TV broadcaster, CBS Sports*
Pete Van Wieren	*Baseball broadcaster for the Atlanta Braves*
Stan Kasten	*Baseball president of the Atlanta Braves*
Leo Mazzone	*Baseball pitching coach for the Atlanta Braves*
Jack Ramsay	*Basketball coach, ESPN pro basketball commentator*
Slick Watts	*Basketball player*
Bob Pettit	*Basketball player*
Curly Neal	*Basketball player with the Harlem Globetrotters*

Nate Thurman	*Basketball player in the Hall of Fame*
Red Auerbach	*Basketball coach and general manager of the Boston Celtics*
Edwin Moses	*Hurdler, won 4 gold medals*
Jesse Owens	*Track star, won 4 gold medals*
Dick Button	*Figure skating world champion, won 2 gold medals*
Bud Collins	*Tennis TV commentator*
Wayne Huizenga	*Owner of professional sport teams*

Bald-Headed Men of America

The wonderful hairitage of shining stars past and present is honored by the Bald-Headed Men of America, the No-Hair Club for Men. Founded in 1973 by John T. Capps III, its purpose is to help make those who lack hair feel good about going bald and to have some fun and build pride in having a chrome dome.

With a heart of gold and a funny bone the size of a walrus, Mr. Capps says that laughter and acceptance are the only real cures for baldness. "I'm not going to lose any hair over it, and I don't want you to either," he says with a smile that lights up the room.

After attending their annual Bald Is Beautiful Convention, humor writer Erma Bombeck reported, "You'll laugh your hair off. While at the convention I had strong feelings of deja vu. I've diapered a lot of babies in my life, and being here brought back a lot of memories!"

For membership and convention information visit the Bald-Headed Men of America Web site at http://members.aol.com/BaldUSA or contact them at:

Bald-Headed Men of America
102 Bald Drive
Morehead City, NC 28557
Tel: (919) 726-1855
Fax: (919) 726-6061

It's more important to have a twinkle in
your eye and a smile on your face.
People remember what's in your heart
longer than what's on your head.
— *John T. Capps III*

4

Baldness Increases Your Face Value: The Advantages of Being Bald

Millions are discovering the dozens of perks that accompany an abundance of scalp. When it comes to increased pleasure, losing your locks is like going from rags to riches—from the comb to the honeycomb.

As you read over the numerous advantages of baldness, allow yourself to deepen in appreciation for the many opportunities you have by simply donning a tailored top.

Time and monetary advantages

- You save valuable time. Men with hair spend an average of 3 days a year with the hair dryer and brush and getting it just right and styling and combing it every time they go to the john.

- You can shampoo in seconds with a washcloth.

- It's low maintenance. You save an average of $326.92 a year by not getting haircuts or purchasing shampoo, combs, brushes, and other hair-care products.

- You do not need hair spray, which by the way, has been used to kill cockroaches.

Relational advantages

- When resting your head on your mate's shoulder your hair will never tickle your loved one's nose.

- Women smile at you in appreciation because they've heard that bald men have more testosterone than other men and thus are more virile.

- There are cranial G-spots all over the top of the bald head. It's a matter of pleasurable discovery.

- Your bald head is very tactile. Women love to rub it—it reminds them of a baby's bottom and all things smooth and round.

Physical advantages

- You never have a bad hair day.

- It's neat and wrinkle-free.

- Being bald is clean, and cleanliness is next to godliness.

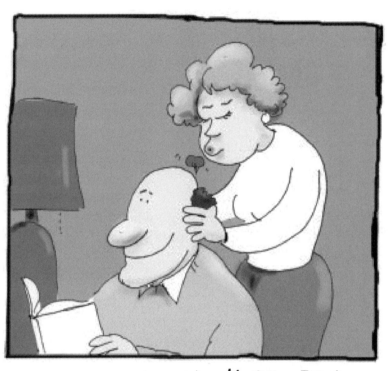

CRANIAL NUDITY – MORE OPEN
SPACE TO CARESS!

Physical advantages (cont)

- It opens up more space for face painting.
- It's an accurate temperature gauge.
- No more cowlicks and never a hair out of place.
- Indoors, you're the first to know the location of the air-conditioning ducts.
- Your hair will never flatten out again after wearing hats.
- Now you can get a total-body tan from head to toe.
- Unlike losing your teeth, going bald is painless and silent.
- You are the first one to know where the cobwebs are while walking on mountain trails.
- Your comb will no longer get tangled up with other things in your pocket.
- A clean head on a fit body enhances the symmetrical skeletal structure of the human form.
- A bald head is soothing and relaxing. When stressed, rubbing your head approximates a cranial massage.
- It's your body's way of getting rid of excess protein.
- You'll have less hair to cut if you go into the military.

Business advantages

- Shaving it all off gives you a unique and distinctive look.

- It reflects clean living and no faking.

- It gives you an honest look that covers up many faults.

- People are more apt to remember you if you're bald.

- When competing you'll always be a head, although it may be a close shave.

- A rolling stone gathers no boss, does not pay rent, and doesn't care because momentum is what it wants to gather.

Social advantages

- You feel a natural skinship with other bald men.

- You'll never get hair in your soup again—unless it's rabbit soup.

- Talking about your cranial coconut is a great icebreaker when you meet people.

- You can have lots of fun with barbers and hair stylists. For instance, you can ask the stylist, "Excuse me, I'd like to get an estimate on your Trac II Casper Cut."

- You'll never have the hair pulled over your eyes.

Social advantages (cont)

- You don't have to go on a vacation to let your hair down.

- You will never be hairied.

- Whenever a problem arises, you'll never lose any hair over it.

God on Baldness

You have been invited to a question-and-answer evening with God, who in this situation takes the form of an older bald man with brilliant silver hair on the sides. It is a time to clear the air on the topic of cranial expansion. You are joined by other bald(ing) men of varying ages along with several men, women, and children who love them.

God: Good evening. I have come here tonight because nobody else is willing to talk candidly about hair addiction and dome denudation. My God (that's Me), hair ranks right up there with money, food, and sex when it comes to emotionally charged issues. In fact, hair addiction is bigger than all these addictions put together! I'm telling you right now, there should be Hair Addicts Anonymous meetings going on in every city and town across the world until this fixation is finally rooted out. Tonight we are going to bring this taboo topic of conversation right out in the open. Does anyone have any questions?

Woman: Yes, Lord, I was wondering why you allowed men to go bald in the first place when you could've arranged it so that all of them kept their hair for a lifetime.

God: Bald men save me a lot of time. Since every hair on their head is counted, I have less work to do when they die—less book-keeping. If everyone had hair I wouldn't get any sleep at all!

Actually, bald men are part of my beautification plan for the human race. Imagine how dull life would be if everyone had hair on their heads. A hairy head is not better than a bald head; it's just different.

Woman: My balding husband keeps telling me that there must be a reason for why he is losing his hair.

God: Balding men are one of my best metaphors. They are living proof that everything is temporary, constantly changing, and will eventually pass away. Everything, including the sun, has a limited life span. My hope is that after we talk here tonight, by just looking at a bald man you will be reminded that love is the *only* thing that is eternal. Everything else, including hair, fades with the passing of time and isn't worth holding on to even for a second!

Bald man: So there's a pearl hidden inside the shell of every loss?

God: Yes. Without loss, you see, life would be very boring and there would be no forward movement or growth at all. Allowing people to experience loss is one of my greatest gifts, because it forces them to move and grow and develop in positive ways. It calls them to reassess what's really important in their lives, to change their thinking and beliefs, and to do things they've never done before.

Whoa! We're gettin' pretty serious here. Anybody heard a good bald joke lately?

Smiling Bald Man: What do you call two fleas on top of a bald head?

God: I don't know. What?

Man: Homeless.

God: Now we're getting somewhere. Laughter is one of my very best inventions. It sure beats frowning and taking things so seriously.

Man:	Yes, humor definitely heals. I feel so great after a good belly laugh.
God:	I am laughter. I am a sense of humor. I mean, who else could create a moon that looks like a bald guy? There he is in the night sky with his glowing curvaceous crest for all to see. The bald moon arising. I am a fungi [fun guy], a comedian, and trying to get people to enjoy my message and not get so hung up on every little word. There's one big word that sums it all up: LOVE. That's it folks—nothing more, nothing less. Love, God, Spirit, and all similar names are talking about the same thing.
Bald man:	Are you saying that since everything comes and goes that we shouldn't take anything, like hair loss, too seriously?
God:	Yes. Hair, like everything we tend to cling to for our source of identity is strictly a passing fancy. Along with your looks, adornments, and admiration from others, your beliefs, morals, feelings, thoughts, desires, and dreams all go at the moment of death.
	Everything you presently look to for your source of happiness comes and goes like the wind. Everything is transitory, in a constant state of flux, and will go the way

of all animate and inanimate objects. When your final curtain call arrives, you will be impelled to let go of absolutely everything. Therefore, love, become love, and learn the art of letting go while alive.

Child: Are there barbershops in heaven?

God: What do you think?

Child: No, but I think there are some bird barbers there.

God: Why do you say that?

Child: Well, somebody has to clip the wings, don't they?

God: What is the one thing that baldness cures?

Child: I don't know. What?

God: Dandruff. It's an advantage of baldness that most people overlook entirely. Would you like to hear a story?

Children: Sure!

God: A man with three hairs on his head walked into the barbershop and sat down in the chair. He told the barber, "Give me a trim and part it on the side." The barber took the scissors and went clip, clip, clip. Then he took his comb and parted it on the side and one of the hairs went "bing!" and fell right off.

The man sighed and said, "Just part it down the middle." The barber combed it over like he instructed and another hair went "bing!" and fell right off. Exasperated, the man sat there for a few moments and said, "Oh, just leave it in a mess."

Woman: Why do so many men spend millions of dollars every year just to have more hair on their heads?

God: They tend to identify hair with who they are, and thus every time a few hairs go down the sink, they feel like a bit of themselves is going down the drain too. Of course, they are not their hair, but they don't realize that yet.

Some want hair for career reasons, while others don't have the confidence to date without some straw on the nest. What I want all balding men to know is that it's the amount of love in their hearts that counts and not what they have or don't have on top. Hair is nothing more than a protein like fingernails and toenails, and is not worthy of being worshipped at all. Let hair, not life, go down the drain and let the bald head reign!

Here's a story I heard recently that speaks

to this point.

Bob and Jim were avid Chicago Cubs baseball fans and attended all the games they could. It was their love of the great American pastime that brought them together. One day while eating peanuts and sipping the foam off the tops of their beers, Bob noticed something different about Jim's head.

"What's different about your head, Jim? It seems like you've got more hair up there."

"Well," Jim confessed, "I've had a few hair transplant treatments done."

"I'm shocked," Bob gulped. "That's like putting astro turf on Wrigley Field! I mean, it's *au naturel* or not at all, baby!"

Friend of a
bald man: Why did you choose to speak to us tonight with a bald head?

God: I simply wanted to demonstrate that being bald is not a liability. It does not in *any* way limit your capacity to love, work, play, or laugh. In fact, your bald head is a perfect vehicle for a lot of funny material. You can get a lot of smileage out of it. The only thing that limits you is your mind. If

45

you think that being bald is a bad thing, then you will feel miserable and have less positive energy to give to your family, relationships, and work.

Like turning on a light switch in a dark room, all you have to do is change the way you think about it and then ACT like being bald is a perfectly fine way to be. The more you USE your head for fun and see the grins you elicit from people wherever you go, the more you will grow to accept and appreciate your head as it is. You need to change not only the way you think about it, but what you do with it as well.

Balding man: Some women tend to place great importance on men having hair.

God: Any woman who places importance on hair in a man when there are so many more important qualities to consider is as shallow as a lake in the Mojave desert. What'll it be, a man with a heart full of love or a head full of hair? Everybody goes bald eventually—love lasts forever.

Anybody got a good story before we close here tonight?

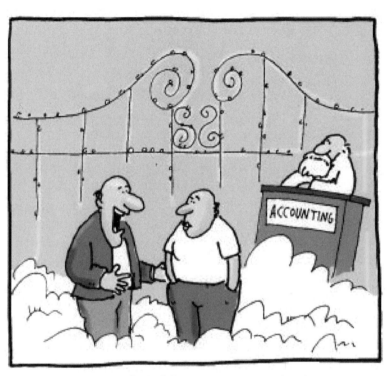

SINCE EVERY HAIR ON OUR HEADS IS COUNTED, WE SHOULD GET RIGHT IN!

Wife of a
bald man: A man was driving down a country road when he ran over a rabbit that had dashed blindly out in front of his car. He got out of the vehicle and was grieving over the dead rabbit when another man came upon the scene.

"What's the matter?" the man asked.

"I just killed this rabbit and I feel awful about it," he answered.

"I can fix that," the passerby commented. He took a small bottle of liquid out of his pocket and poured it on the dead rabbit. In a few seconds, the rabbit got up on all fours and started walking down the street. About fifty yards away the rabbit turned to the two men and waved at them with his right paw. Fifty yards later he did the same thing.

"What did you put on the rabbit?" the man asked in amazement.

"Hare restorer and permanent wave," he replied.*

God: Laughter makes the world go 'round. So laugh, grow hair, love, lose hair, let go, and go bald. Good night.

* Every effort has been made to find the author of this story. If you are the creator of this story please contact us and we will include your name in future editions.

6

What Bald Golfers Know

"Give me my golf clubs, the fresh air and a beautiful woman as a partner—and you can have the clubs and the fresh air."
—George Burns

The next time you hit the links with your friends or are just sitting around talking golf, you can dig into this bagful of 48 witty things to say that will establish you as the head of your group.

Bald golfers know that . . .

- Grass doesn't grow on a busy street or cart path.

- From tee to green only the fringe can be seen.

- There are no mulligans ("do-overs") once you lose your hair. "Now you have it; now you don't" is God's irreversible little joke.

- The real "Skins" game is played by baldheaded golfers only.

- Baldies are guaranteed to start the Seniors Tour with a clean slate.

Bald golfers know that . . .

- Combing the rough over the dogleg left will attract fewer women golfers to the course.
- Bald cypress trees thrive at Pebble Beach.
- There is one type of birdie that golfers call regal, Which is none other than the baldheaded eagle.
- The slickest way to drive a green is in a golf cart with bald tires.
- If only one bald man is there, a sound is still made by a tiger in the woods.
- Although they have the same number of shafts as hair-full players, bald players will always have fewer strokes.
- Even if they score high, they always come away with a good *round*.
- Men with hairpieces are usually trying to improve their lie.
- They are on every leader board when it comes to sex appeal.
- For women, the bald head is a fairway to heaven.
- The British are Open to Harry and the Non-Hairy alike.
- There is no fair way. What once was fuzz eventually becomes the fuzz that was.

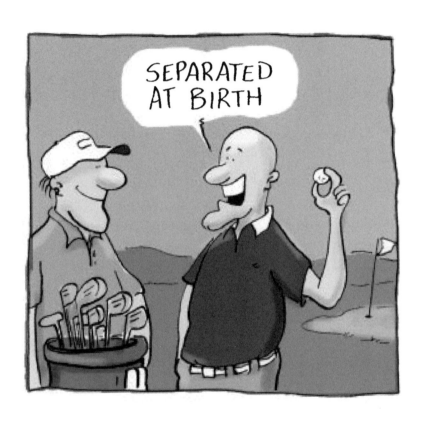

Bald golfers know that . . .

- You can iron out all difficulties by simply shooting straight.

- While bald men may not make every cut, they'll always come out a head.

- Like dimples on a golf ball, the bald head provides many spots to kiss and caress.

- Hairless golfers will never get sand in their hair when blasting out of a trap.

- They are Pavin' the way for more future stars with glistening orbs.

- Bald heads are "Taylor made" by God.

- When it comes to hair, you don't get a second drop.

- Baldies are merely a chipping wedge off the old block.

- Hitting the links is time better spent than combing the locks.

- You can get teed off after shooting an 80 at St. Andrews, with or without hair.

- For bald men, winning any major is a crowning glory.

- Once your hair is gone, all you can say is, "Shanks for the memories."

Bald golfers know that . . .

- A water hole is but a reflecting pool for waveless wonders to gaze delightedly upon their image.
- A baldface lie is when your ball lands cleanly atop any smooth surface such as a road, path, drainage cover, or someone's back porch.
- Putting their Pate-in-place is a Daly task for most tour players.
- They'll never end up in the tall grass.
- It would be Strange if Curtis went bald or if Andy's hair went North.
- They never have to comb their hair before TV interviews.
- Big Bertha loves bald guys.
- Hair will never fall into their eyes when putting.
- Artificial turf of any kind is a turnoff to discerning women.
- Graphite shaft implants just might be the hair-raising technology of the future.
- God is the architect of their course and their personal greenskeeper.
- There are no Pebbles on their Beach.
- By driving a Cadillac they'll always have their own personal caddie.

Bald golfers know that . . .

- Tees for two are quite common with virile crested men.

- For men growing in wisdom, age, and understanding, being bald is par for the course.

- By not puttering around with hair, they have more time to read greens and good novels.

- Divots can be replaced but a good bald man cannot.

- Anyway you slice it, when your hair begins to fade, you'll never become a hooker just to compensate or to increase your draw.

Hair Ye, Hair Ye, What Is Thy Purpose?

Hair: One of the cylindrical, often pigmented filaments characteristically growing from the epidermis of a mammal.

Bald: Unadorned, undisguised, honest and open, as in "the bald truth." Bare (syn): devoid of amplification or adornment, removal of what is superfluous. Naked (syn): a state of nature, of simple beauty.

Every species will do what it has to do in order to survive. For instance, when the first species of lizards came out of the ocean and discovered that gills were no longer needed, they gradually shed their gills and evolved into a land reptile. Adaptation was necessary to survive. Crushing molars and strong mandibles, for example, were once needed by our earliest ancestors for grinding coarse vegetation and cracking nuts. These were eventually replaced when smaller teeth and jaws became necessary for eating meat.

For cavemen and their offspring, hair served a very useful purpose. It helped keep them warm and protected from the elements. As they trudged through forests, hair was a buffer between skin and limb. It prevented burning by the scorching sun and cushioned the scalp from falling objects. It discouraged insects looking for an open space, shielded the pearly pate from biting winds, and acted as a sponge for water, allowing vision to be clearer while hunting and clearing paths. In short, hair was necessary for survival.

In time, as our brain power and consciousness increased, head coverings and homes of all shapes and sizes were made to keep the head warm and protect it from the elements. Suntan lotions and sunscreens also took the place of hair as further safeguards against the elements. Whereas early man depended on hair all over his body as a protection, people today use clothing, shelter, and hats as body and pate preservation shields.

Our earliest ancestors did not have these protections. They needed their cylindrical and often pigmented filaments to prevent a prunelike appearance that could've turned off their feminine cavemates and prevented future generations from being born. Hair was a necessity, a sine qua non for staying alive.

Today, however, like so many things that were once considered indispensable, the mane is on the wane. It is now quite evident that hair serves one primary, albeit unnecessary, purpose: ornamentation. The decorated dome links us with our Neanderthal brothers, whose total body hirsuteness was the undisputed style of the day. Cavewomen were wild about Hairy. But what about the body of the future? Scientists tell us that our bodies in years to come will have less and less hair.

According to them, the images of advanced bald aliens that we see in science fiction movies are not far from the truth.

Despite this natural evolutionary trend from hair to bare, many still follow in the footsteps of those who viewed hair as synonymous with being virile, masculine, and strong. Samson, for instance, believed that strength was somehow connected to his hair and that its loss would cause him to be ineffective in battle. Likewise, Julius Caesar found himself desperately seeking strands for fear that his follicular fallout would bring him disfavor.

Since then, on the heels of Yul Brynner, Telly Savalas, Lou Gossett Jr., and Michael Jordan, thousands of soldiers, athletes, and public figures have proven that power, manliness, and style can be embodied in the bald.

In the last hair analysis, we find that hair is no longer functionally imperative to our well-being nor necessary to attract a desirable mate. While hair still provides some protection when hitting our peaks on chandeliers, open cabinet doors, and low entryways, its protective purpose is now realistically limited to a few times a year. As we dispensed with hood ornaments on cars because they no longer enhanced the aesthetic quality of the vehicle, we can now let our top down, have fun with our threadbare epidermis, and simply enjoy the ride. By letting nature naturally remove what is superfluous, we stand open-ended to a bright and shining future.

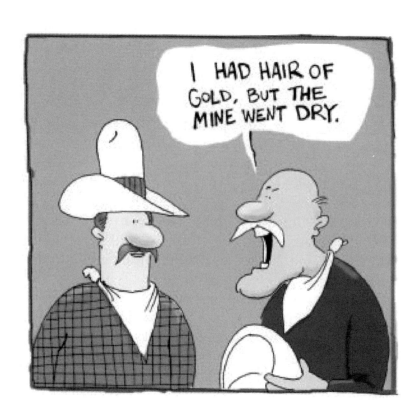

Bald Trivia II

When you have guests over, it's fun to play trivia games. If you want the game to last longer, you may want to start with "Bald Trivia I" from the first book, *Bald Men Always Come Out on Top,* and then finish with "Bald Trivia II." By using the voice of a game show host you will help set a fun and friendly competitive atmosphere. Have someone keep score as you go along and offer a prize for the person with the most correct responses.

1. Name the hairless author and publisher whose name appears on cake boxes worldwide.
    — Duncan Hines

2. Name the British playwright who said the following quote later made famous by President John F. Kennedy, "Some people see things as they are and ask 'Why?' I dream of things that never were and ask 'Why not?' "
    — George Bernard Shaw

3. Name a famous bald Italian dictator.

— Benito Mussolini

4. What causes a bald head?

— A lack of hair

5. This bald singer and songwriter wrote the song *Fire and Rain*.

— James Taylor

6. What famous bald comedic actor said, "I was in the hospital recently and took a turn for the nurse."

— W. C. Fields

7. This famous Russian composer wrote the ballet *The Nutcracker*.

— Tchaikovsky

8. Name two bald cartoon characters.

— Ziggy, Henry, Linus, Mr. Magoo, Elmer Fudd

9. Known as the greatest circus man on earth, this legendary bald promoter had associates that included a giant elephant and a tiny English folk hero.

— P. T. Barnum

10. What is round and soft and really fun to play with?

— Your favorite bald head

11. What do Sun Yat-sen and Chiang Kai-shek have in common?

— They are both men, bald, and Chinese political leaders. Any of these answers is correct.

12. What is the traditional ceremony for a Jewish man who is losing his hair?

— A baldmitzvah

13. What was the name of the original hairless host on the weekly TV show "Candid Camera"?

— Allen Funt

14. This leading French man of letters wrote

about the 1755 earthquake in Lisbon, Portugal, that killed 30,000 people in his witty and satirical attack on optimism entitled *Candide*.
— François-Marie Arouet de Voltaire

15. What is the perfect cure for dandruff?
    — Baldness

16. This American doctor is the author of *Love, Medicine, and Miracles*.
    — Dr. Bernie Siegel

17. Name three bald comedians.
    — Don Rickles, Dom DeLuise, Leo Gallagher, W. C. Fields, Harpo Marx, Zero Mostel

18. What is the bald man's favorite flower?
    — Twolips, placed affectionately on top of his head

19. This Russian-born composer is most famous for his ballets *The Rite of Spring* and *The Firebird*, his opera *Oedipus Rex*, and his chamber piece *The Soldier's Tale*.
    — Igor Stravinsky

20. What famous ventriloquist had a sky-clad dome?
   — Edgar Bergen

21. What do you call 288 hairs on top of a
    man's head?
   — Too gross

22. This American industrialist, philanthropist, and
    owner of a steel empire, believed that no man
    should die wealthy and had a contempt for
    inheritance as a way of attaining wealth.
   — Andrew Carnegie

23. Simon and Garfunkel had such musical hits as
    Bridge Over Troubled Waters, *Mrs. Robinson*, and
    Scarborough Fair. Which one of them has a long
    forehead?
   — Art Garfunkel

24. What was the name of the first bald Native
    American chief?
   — Chief Bigface

25. What was the name of his beloved son?
   — Little Hare

26. This bald Dane with hardly any mane is famous for his composition of children's fairy tales.
    — Hans Christian Anderson

27. In the group Crosby, Stills, and Nash, which one of them was as hairless as a drum?
    — David Crosby

28. This Prussian statesman, sometimes called the "Iron Chancellor," was the architect of German unification and the arbiter of European power politics in the second half of the nineteenth century. He also had a ship named after him.
    — Otto Von Bismarck

29. What famous American architect was as smooth as glass on his dome?
    — Frank Lloyd Wright

30. This English poet became established as the most popular poet of the Victorian era with his poems "In Memoriam" and "The Princess."
    — Alfred, Lord Tennyson

31. Name one former bald U.S. Secretary of State.
    — Alexander Haig Jr., Dean Rusk

32. What are the three ways a man can wear his hair?
    — Parted, unparted, departed

33. What is the name of the bald Russian writer who wrote one of the most well known novels ever written—*War and Peace*?
    — Count Leo Tolstoy

34. Name a famous Olympic track star who won four gold medals while running topless around the track.
    — Edwin Moses, Jesse Owens

35. What is the bald man's favorite golf tournament?
    — The Skins game

36. Name two races of men who are less likely to go bald.
    — Asian, African American, Native American

37. Name one professional bald hockey player.
    — Mark Messier, Roger Crozier, Lorne

Henning, Bobby Shehan, Howie Morenz,
Jacques Lemaire, Donnie Marshall,
Dennis Hull, Dave Ballone,
Wayne Cashman, Billy Rey, Ivan Johnson,
Jack Crawford, Bill White, or Gary Bergman.

38. What highly intelligent English poet was married
to Elizabeth Barrett Browning?
— Robert Browning

39. What are the four kinds of hair?
— In, Thin, Fuzz, and Was

40. What do Red Auerbach and Rick Majerus have
in common?
— They are both bald basketball coaches.

41. Name a bald baseball player who played
before 1985.
—Harmon Killebrew, Gaylord Perry, Yogi Berra,
Vic Power, Chris Chambliss, Sal Bando,
Enos Slaughter, Warren Spahn, Cy Young,
Luis Tiant, Rick Reuschel, Eddie Matthews.

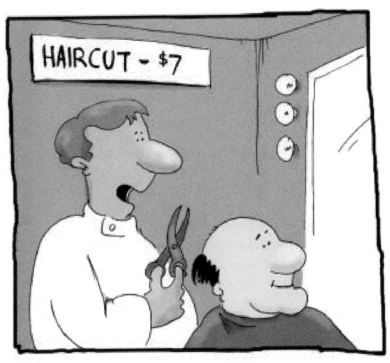

IT'LL BE FIVE DOLLARS TO FIND IT, AND TWO DOLLARS TO CUT IT.

42. What bald man was president of North Vietnam from 1945 to 1969?
    — Ho Chi Minh

43. True or false? Ours is the true religion.
    — Ah-hah, you tricked 'em! After the laughter subsides, move right along to the next question.

44. What do you call a discarded toupee?
    — A throw rug

45. Who was the first baldheaded cowboy in motion pictures who had a wide part in "The Magnificent Seven?"
    — Yul Brynner

46. What famous Greek bald man is known as the "father of medicine" and once declared from personal experience that pigeon droppings on the scalp was a disadvantage of baldness?
    — Hippocrates

47. At least one man on this planet has grown a full head of hair after using a hair-growth medication like Minoxidil. True or false?
    — False

48. Who was the first baldheaded baseball manager to finish first?
    — Leo Durocher

49. What type of hair lotion did the bald ESPN college basketball analyst Dick Vitale use when he used to have hair?
    — Vitalis

50. This daughter of Henry VIII and Queen of England was bald and wore a red wig, the color of her original hair. Who was she?
    — Elizabeth I, the Virgin Queen

51. Who was the first baldheaded man in space?
    — John Glenn

52. In the elections of 1952 and 1956, what two baldheaded men ran head to head for the presidency of the United States?
— Dwight D. Eisenhower and Adlai Stevenson

53. Who was the first baldheaded man to walk on the moon?
— Edwin "Buzz" Aldrin

54. Sy Sperling is the founder and president of "The Hair Club for Men" and also one of its members. What did he do before becoming America's Rug King?
— He was a carpet salesman. Thus, before he sold rugs, he sold rugs.

55. Only one business offers a 100% guarantee that baldness can be cured? What is that business?
— The tire retreading business

The Eagle Has Landed
Societal Acceptance of Baldness
Close at Hand

Once the eagle lands, it has been foretold, men and women everywhere will finally pay due reverence to the cranius rotundus. At that time, the dynamic dome will be recognized as the reflecting pool of wisdom that it naturally is. The majestic, magical, and towering Eagle has been expected for centuries. Men and women have been gazing skyward, wondering if the eagle they see is the "One" who is to come. Many birds of excellence have set down their feet on the hallowed ground of earth, but only one has landed, drawing the attention of millions across the planet.

From the 1950s to the dawn of the new millennia, it has been primarily a hairy road. During this period our societal value makers have prized hair beyond rational explanations. Entertainers, politicians, and athletes, until recent times, have conveyed the message that hair was equal to good looks and good luck and was the necessary accoutrement to dating, mating, and finding a desirable job.

Hair, or filaments designed primarily to protect and catch dirt and sweat, has become the single most fussed-over area of our bodies. Billions of dollars a year are spent to clean, condition, curl, color, straighten, mousse, and gel locks, and to try to put an end to trichoptilosis—split ends (the frizzies). While we've been told that personality and being true to one's values were what really counted, the bottom line has consistently been that plumage was number one and the peek-a-boo do number two.

In the 1950s, glossy General Dwight D. Eisenhower ("Ike") became the hair apparent to the presidential throne. However, in this Age of Hair, the thirty-fourth president of the United States was not the role model for heads of state nor states of head. There were no teenagers or military enlistees proclaiming "I want to be like Ike" or choosing to go one step beyond the crew cut or the G.I. (Government Issue) hairstyle. Although a significant leader of his time, he was not the Regal Eagle who was to come.

Phil Silvers and Jimmy Durante were among the decade's best comedians, but they held no influence on the coiffing practices of the time. Likewise, Red Auerbach, winner of nine NBA titles as coach of the Boston Celtics, did not soar to the head of the most influential list. Although the Dalai Lama has thousands of bald Buddhist devotees, he has made little impact on the greater hair-attached world.

Although not the first to shave his head, Academy Award-winning Yul Brynner brought baldness out of the closet. Through his powerful role as the King of Siam in "The King and I," he became a symbol of male sexuality and charm. Was *he* the long-awaited Eagle? Despite his reign of popularity, lasting for many years, Brynner failed to spark a Yul tide of waveless followers. His candle grew dim over time and effected no increase in the number of men choosing to shave their heads. Elvis Presley, on the other hand, clearly led the way in the image and hair department of the '50s. He was not only the undisputed king of rock and roll, but also the full-cropped king of coif.

The '60s showed off long locks from the Beatles to hippies in an era when trust of elders, self-discipline, and crew cuts reached an all-time low. Longer hairstyles dominated during the time period as Beattle Mane-ia swept the world. With hair being the decade's defining trait, long-haired rock groups appeared everywhere, shaking their locks to the beat of a new wave of music. The popular musical "Hair" fit right in with the focus of the time. Hair was the way you proved to the world that you were a "cool" or "groovy" person. Elvis was still idolized during this period, mostly by people watching him shake, rattle, and roll on the big screen.

During this period and for decades following, Joe Garagiola broke the hair barrier without de-balding or giving in to the "you oughtta get a toupee" pressure. He was the first hairless game show host and the first bald man to anchor the Today Show. And every Saturday afternoon was made brighter and happier because Joe Garagiola called the play-by-play on TV's baseball game of the week.

He was a dome alone in a hairied world, where bald(ing) baseball players would do anything to avoid losing their helmets when sliding into a base. He bared all at a time when bald(ing) players would often stay in the dugout rather than remove their hats for the playing of the "Star Spangled Banner." While enhancing the enjoyment of baseball for fans everywhere, this witty, lovable, and handsome man was not to become the guru of glossy globes. However, by standing firm amidst a panoply of hairy-pated public personas, he became a bulwark for baldness and the cornerstone for the future bald hall of fame.

The '70s brought hair transplants more prominently on the scene with the hope that the hair would take root and help remove some of the pain of hairlessness. Despite Telly "Kojak" Savalas hitting his peak in the '70s, long hair was still the style of the day. This shaved-head icon of masculinity appeared on his top-rated "Kojak" television series for five years running. Despite the fact that many saw him as "The Eagle," his prominence was not enough to inspire others to follow in his hairless wake.

By sporting a shaved, bald head for decades, one man made significant headway in making the bald head popular and acceptable. The image and power of his shaved head in the movie *An Officer and a*

Gentleman, remains etched in the consciousness of all who witnessed his performance. Likewise, his portrayal of a wise, intelligent, and compassionate slave in *Roots* showed the world that a bald black actor could do it all. He is the Oscar-winning Louis Gossett Jr.

The first shaved-head professional basketball player of the '70s was Slick Watts, whose trademark headband made him immediately recognizable on any court in session. The number of watts that gleamed off his head during an average game is not known. Despite being renowned and well-received by fans in Seattle, New Orleans, and Houston, his "air style" did not start a topless trend. However, he was truly a precursor to the "One" who was to come.

During the early '70s a talented, funny, and dedicated bald man appeared on the scene. After being turned down for a job because his round crown did not fit the company's image, John T. Capps III founded an organization called The Bald-Headed Men of America. With his Topless Club for men he seeks to eliminate the vanity associated with hair loss, and to instill pride and dignity in accepting baldness. Through his yearly Bald Is Beautiful Convention, he has played a wide part in putting baldness on the map of acceptability. Although not visible enough to be hairalded as the "Eagle Par Excellence," this cross between Mr. Clean and the moon has been a bright light for baldies everywhere.

The Upjohn Company, who came out with a hair-growth medication in the late 1970s called Minoxidil, appeared to answer the need for something to grow

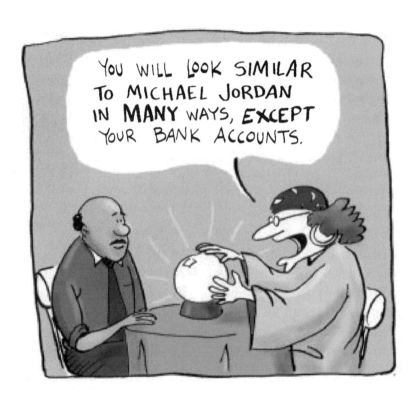

hair without having to get a surgical transplant or don a toupee or weave. Originally, Minoxidil was used as a means of treating high blood pressure, but some of its users noticed that as a side-effect it grew hair on the tips of their noses. Fascinated with the possibilities, the company experimented with a liquid variation called Rogaine Topical Solution that was applied directly to the scalp. It was eventually approved by the Food and Drug Administration and worked best for young men (especially on the crowns of their heads) and those who hadn't lost much hair.

In the early 1980s addiction to hair was still the sine qua non for being sexually attractive. However, it was also a time when more and more men were letting their hair down in the form of toupees and hair weaves. Although thin was more in than in previous decades, the thought of acquiring more hair without going under the knife continued to fascinate thousands. Thus, many still turned to Minoxidil in hopes of resurrecting a few forlorn follicles. In the end it was nowhere near the magic elixir that people hoped it would be.

As transplanters approached the time for new plugs and an oil change in the late '80s, many others declared that "enough was enough" and that being natural was the preferable way to go. More and more started to say "no" to hair additions and realized that hair did not make the man. Men could lose their hair, unlike Samson of old, without losing their outer and inner strength.

Although it was in no way a time of total head

liberation for men, it was a moment when many of them took stock of what celebrities were doing with their pates. Stars like Michael Keaton, Bruce Willis, and Bill Murray showed men everywhere that one could be both bankable and balding.

Other bald men began making headway in a variety of fields. The esteemed skin abundant astronaut John Glenn, for example, was shining forth in the Senate, while bald basketball star Kareem Abdul Jabbar was on his way to becoming the most prolific scorer in the history of the game. Although not able to swing society away from its obsession with hair, these men, along with many others, helped set the stage for the nude awakening in the '90s. They prepared the dome-shaped dais for the Esteemed Eagle, the Defender of Light.

Soaring to unbelievable heights on the foundation built by Brynner, Watts, Jabbar, Garagiola, Savalas, Capps, and Lou Gosset Jr., the Chicago Bull's superstar, Michael Jordan, came on the scene. He was clearly THE EAGLE, the long-awaited classy chassis with no fringe on top. Choosing the Trac II home version "Casper Cut," he single-headedly made it okay for anyone to be bald. He created a new headstyle that can be seen on heads around the world.

Thousands of "I want to be like Mike" athletes, fans, and fellow NBA players shaved their heads as a sign of special skinship with arguably the best basketball player of all time. They were imitating Michael like congregations of worshipers seeking to take on the characteristics of their deity. It was as if his new pruned pinnacle enhanced his aerodynamic capacity even more as he flew gracefully to the basket.

Fellow basketball greats Charles Barkley, Shaquille O'Neal, and a slew of other NBA stars have come clean along with many other professional players. As more and more of these athletes are baring it all and becoming comfortable in their own skin, receding men are seeing with their own eyes that shedding one's hair does not diminish one's appeal. On the contrary. The fact is that right now millions of very satisfied women are in love with happily hairless men across the globe.

Skin is more in now than ever before and shows no signs of shrinking in popularity. Rockers, actors, athletes, teenagers and executives are playing the hair game on a clear field. Some are doing it to defeat their hairline before their locks head completely north. Others are going bald by design. History has led us to this polished point in time. The peerless pates of such giants as Shakespeare, Darwin, Churchill, Tolstoy, and Gandhi have paved the way for men like Sean Connery, John Glenn, Montel Williams, Dick Vitale, Lou Gossett Jr., Stephen R. Covey, and The Eagle, Air Jordan himself. These and thousands of others, known and unknown, stand as models of maneless magnificence, proving that hair is not needed to make a positive contribution in the world.

Societal acceptance of baldness is close at hand. The man with the leonine mane no longer sits alone on the throne of masculinity. From entertainers, musicians, writers, and world leaders to politicians, sport figures, and spiritual giants, bald heads are smoothing cities and towns everywhere showing that there's no place quite like dome. The spate of bald pates is swelling, with more than 55 million 40-plus baby boomers adding "no-frills" beauty to the landscape. These intelligent, creative, and powerful men have laid bare the truth that hair is simply not needed to live a happy, love-full, and successful life. One day soon society will make the relatively short leap to the other side of hair. At that time, men and women globally will celebrate baldness as a perfectly wonderful and natural way to be.

Dome Improvement: A New Vocabulary for the Emerging Bald Paradigm

It is time to let sleeping dogmas lie and to raise our thoughts and speech about the bald head to new levels of respectability. Now is the moment to move from hairbrained ideas to ribald humor about what cranial nudity really means. As millions of men are proudly and voluntarily donning the dynamic dome, the time is ripe to change the way we think and speak about the sacred space known as our head. Out of the mouths of babes comes cereal. But out of the mouths of bald men and those who love them, needs to come a powerful new vocabulary aimed at replacing all the derogatory words formerly used to describe the bald head.

To help change the way people think and speak about the brilliant star on top of our shoulders, we need to correct them whenever they use demeaning names. For instance, when someone says, "Hey, chrome dome!" we need to reply nonreactively, "Excuse me, sir, 'chrome dome' is no longer the appropriate term to use—it has been replaced with 'aerodynamic brow.' I would appreciate your using that term from now on."

Or, if someone calls us "cue ball" or "bowling ball" we need to inform them that these words have been replaced with "sculptured speed bump" and "rolling stone." Let them know that Daniel Webster, who was as bald as a ballerina's armpit, did not include these descriptions when defining "bald" in the dictionary.

It is quite chic nowadays for newspaper and television reporters to use seemingly erudite descriptions for the bald head that are subtly degrading. For instance, when they call us "follicly challenged" or "hair impaired" we need to gently set them straight. "Follicly natural" and "hair free" are the new respectful and politically correct terms to use.

Bald men and those who love them need to stand up for names that affirm the dignity, acceptability, and respectability of bald heads everywhere. Let the new vocabulary begin.

Names used under the old paradigm	Names to be used under the new paradigm
Chrome dome	Aerodynamic brow
Baldy	No-frills beauty
Air head	Sky-clad dome
Cue ball	Sculptured speed bump
Greaseball	Glistening orb

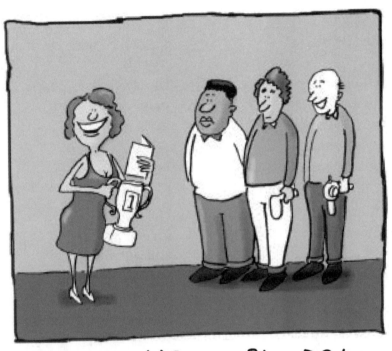

...AND THE NATIONAL BLOW DRYING
CHAMPION IS...

Old paradigm	New paradigm
Crystal ball	Lustrous lamp
Melon head	Round crown
Shinola	Beautiful beaming bean
Mr. Clean	Lean and mean clean machine
Bald head	Classy chassis, pearly pate, clean slate
Bowling ball	Rolling stone
Loss of hair	Cranial nudity
No hair man	Wave of the future
Follicly challenged	Follicly natural
Hair impaired	Hair free
Lightheaded	Free of all entanglements
Bald as a tire	Smooth as a baby's bottom
Shiner	Solar energy panel for a sex machine
Curly	Pruned pinnacle of perfection
Hairy	Dynamic dome
Skinhead	The real skinny
Oh, the glare!	Hail to the sun kissed peak!
Going bald	Starting a second face
Egghead	Wis-dome

Old paradigm	New paradigm
Slick	Barren beacon
Losing hair	The mane on the wane
Coconut head	Curvaceous crest
Bald as a baboon's butt	Bald as a ballerina's armpit
Bald as a coot	Naked as a jay bird
Hairless wonder	Sexy, virile, masculine
Buffed head	Testosterone top

When all is said and done, the quality with which we have loved will stand above all heads and all things temporary as the gauge for a truly successful life.
— *from* Bald Men Always Come Out on Top

The Bald Path: A Smooth Road in a Rocky World

"Don't follow the path. Go where there is no path and begin the trail. When you start a new trail equipped with courage, strength, and conviction, the only thing that can stop you is you."

—Ruby Bridges, civil rights pioneer

The Bald Path is the least expensive, least worrisome, and least painful option to hair loss there is. It is for those who have considered the available options and have chosen to accept their baldness and make the most of it.

Like a rolling stone that gathers no moss, the Bald Path is a declaration of independence from hair. It is about walking free without being attached to anything along the way. Whether it's hair or the thought that hair is necessary to land a beautiful mate, Bald Pathers know that *all* must be released when the final bell tolls. In the end, as always, they realize that it is the quality with which they have loved, not the amount of hair they have on their heads, that is most important. The

Bald Path teaches them that love does not come to them because they have locks or look a certain way, but because they are willing to love—willing to consistently give of their energy and attention to others.

The Bald Path clearly purports that baldness is NOT a problem, but a perfectly fine way to be. Bald Pathers are well aware that since 98.5 percent of all people don't really care if they are bald or not, they should spend *no* time worrying about it themselves. They are well aware that millions of women are attracted to, love, and even prefer baldheaded men, and that no bald(ing) man who dares to love will ever be left out in the relationship department. If he will but care about serving and contributing to the good of others and the world, he will receive love back a hundredfold.

The Bald Path, sculptured by Mother Nature, is lined with acceptance, wisdom, and humor. It is not about trying to be perfect, as if a full head of hair represented the ideal. For Bald Pathers it is about learning to embrace and accept themselves as they are right now. Because no more costly gardeners are needed to trim, shape, and coif their cylindrical filaments, they smile in appreciation.

This is a smooth road because positivity, acceptance, and love are the signposts along the way. It is not made smooth by leveling others or criticizing people who don't think like they do. It is not about putting men down who have hair, or about trying to embarrass and uncover those who wish to go undercover and stay that way. Nor is it about lambasting hair replacement or hair restoration companies or condemning those who opt for either rugs, plugs, drugs, or combovers as their hair loss option of choice. Rather, it is about making others feel good about themselves and being alive.

Members of the Bald Path know that getting new hair will not help them to love themselves or cause them to grow in self-confidence. They understand that it is only by loving their families, friends, and the world that they will feel a sense of connectedness that naturally heals. It is only by loving and giving freely that others will mirror the reflection of love back into their own eyes and hearts. Doing and feeling and living and praying and playing and being with and for others is the foundational value upon which Bald Pathers build their lives.

They realize that changing their mind, not their hairline, is the key to a happier and healthier life. They've learned that by simply changing the way they think about being bald their lives move in a more positive direction. For instance, by turning the mistaken thought that "women are not attracted to baldheaded men" into "I am attractive to many women," they immediately widen the path for others to walk side by side.

Although Bald Pathers may have dropped out on top, they have tuned in to what is most important in life. Rather than covering up in any way, they proclaim a resounding "yes" to accepting what they have and making the most of it. By speaking positively about their bald heads and consciously using them to bring joy into the lives of others, they create a positive and loving energy around them that naturally attracts joy and people with a similar resonance.

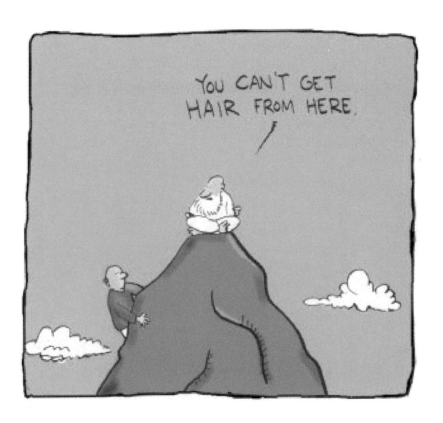

Being bald is a showcase for bedroom eyes.

Index

Mission Statement

Dave Beswick is committed to:

- Serving bald(ing) men.

- Supporting and working with men who are having difficulty with their hair loss.

- Educating parents, mates and friends of bald(ing) men about what these men are going through and how to serve them in sensitive and effective ways.

- Showing men who are happily hairless how to use their heads as a positive asset in order to bring more joy and laughter into the world.

- Teaching men who have come to peace with their heads how to be mentors to younger men who are going through the often painful time of hair loss.

- Helping raise awareness that baldness is not a problem or something negative, but rather a natural and perfectly fine way to be.

- Laughing, loving, and letting go.

Spread Cheer from Ear to Ear

"When we laugh, it lowers our blood pressure, because laughter causes our blood vessels to dilate—and that is certainly better than having them die early."
— Swami Beyondananda, a.k.a. Steve Bhaerman

"A day without laughter is a wasted day. Learn to laugh. No matter what you do, you can do it better with humor. Laughter is the miracle drug you carry with you all day long that costs nothing."
— George Lewis, founder of the
National Laugh Foundation

"Time spent laughing is time spent with the gods."
— Japanese proverb

"He is not a wise man who cannot play the fool on occasion."
— Anonymous

"Hearty laughter is a good way to jog internally without having to go outdoors."
— Norman Cousins

"Humor is a serious thing. I like to think of it as one of our greatest resources, which must be preserved at all costs."
— James Thurber

"A sense of humor is a major defense against minor troubles."
— Mignon McLaughlin

"He who laughs, lasts."
— Mary Pettibone Poole

About the Author

Dave Beswick:

- Was born with cranial peach fuzz on October 30, 1946.

- Dearly loved his German Short Hair dog named Nibs who was easy to wash after finding golf balls at the local course.

- Rooted for bald 49er quarterback Y.A. Tittle and listened to hairless Joe Garagiola announce baseball games.

- Pushed his teenage hairs around to cover up open spaces.

- Mistakenly thought for years that women were only attracted to men with hair and that locks were needed to feel secure, confident, and socially at ease.

- Felt stunned when informed by his dermatologist that he had hand-me-down recessive genes and that every hair on his head was worth two in the brush.

- Was voted "Most likely to recede" at his high school graduation.

- Worked in Alaska where mosquitoes used his head as a landing strip.

- Once considered applying warm cow dung to his scalp to grow hair at the recommendation of a Catholic nun.

- Regularly stood upside down on a backswing to try and get blood flowing to his scalp to stimulate growth—no hair-raising developments occurred.

- Discovered that women were attracted to him and that hair was not necessary to live a happy, love-full, and successful life.

- Entered the Jesuit order and was dispensed from getting a tonsure (the act of shaving the crown of a monk's head) because he already had it naturally.

- Married Janie in an old rustic church near Half Dome in Yosemite National Park.

- Received "The Smoothest Bald Head" award at his 25th high school reunion and the "Kelsey Grammer Look-a-like" award at the Bald-Headed Men of America annual convention.

Additional Information

SPEAKING ENGAGEMENTS

Dave Beswick offers speaking engagements on a variety of topics tailored to the needs of each group. If you want your audiences to have fun, learn something they can practically use in their own lives, and leave inspired for living more fully and joyfully, invite Dave to speak to your group. For a list of topics and to schedule appearances call 1-888-BALD-101 (1-888-225-3101).

BOOKS BY DAVE BESWICK

The following books of positive bald wit and wisdom are for those who are looking into the various options to hair loss and want to consider the advantages of learning to accept what they have and make the most of it. They are also for men who are happily hairless, who appreciate the many fringe benefits of being bald, and who want more slick wit available to them to make people smile from ear to ear. And lastly, they are for those who know or love a baldheaded man and want to give him a quality gift that says, "You're the greatest."

Bald Men Always Come Out on Top—*101 Ways to Use Your Head and Win with Skin*, shows happily hairless men how to have fun with their sleek peaks, what to say when hair-assed, how to enjoy nature head-on, and how to take maximum advantage of their fringe benefits and become empowered as baldheaded men.

Bald Men Never Have a Bad Hair Day—*Wit and Wisdom for Men on the Bald Path*, teaches topless men how baldness increases their face value, what bald golfers know, what God thinks about baldness, and gives them a new positive bald vocabulary and the perspective needed to walk joyfully on the Bald Path.

Bald Men Rise and Shine! shows why bald men get better with age, the many advantages of being bald, the importance of connecting with our roots, how to use our heads to bring joy to others, what bald athletes know, why women give bald(ing) men the go a head, and provides insightful answers to the most frequently asked questions about dealing with hair loss.

Each of these books is available for $9.95 in bookstores and gift stores everywhere or toll free at 1-800-507-2665.

Bald men are capable of great introspection, and when standing under a light, are capable of even greater reflection.

Dear Reader,

Thank you for reading this book. We would like to leave you with a few final thoughts. Peace of mind occurs whenever we are able to accept what is and make the most of it. If you are looking into various options to hair loss, we invite you to consider the advantages of learning to accept your head as it is and make the most of what you have. Without a doubt, it is the least expensive, least worrisome, and least painful option to hair loss there is.

The books in the "Bald Men" series are for those moving towards acceptance and those who are happily hairless either by design or by Mother Nature. They offer over 150 things we can say and do to use our heads in a positive way. Our task is to choose expressions and actions that are comfortable for us to use and then to try them out in a variety of situations.

May you be inspired to take plenty of time to appreciate and enjoy your head as it is. May it be a source of joy for you and those you meet along the way.

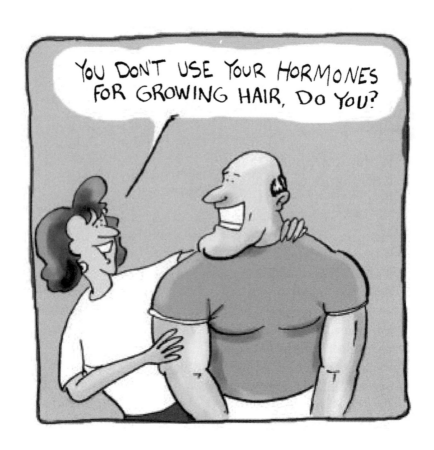